CW01664391

STRESS MANAGEMENT FOR WOMEN

How to Stop Negative Thinking and Control Your Thoughts

Isabel Rose

TABLE OF CONTENTS

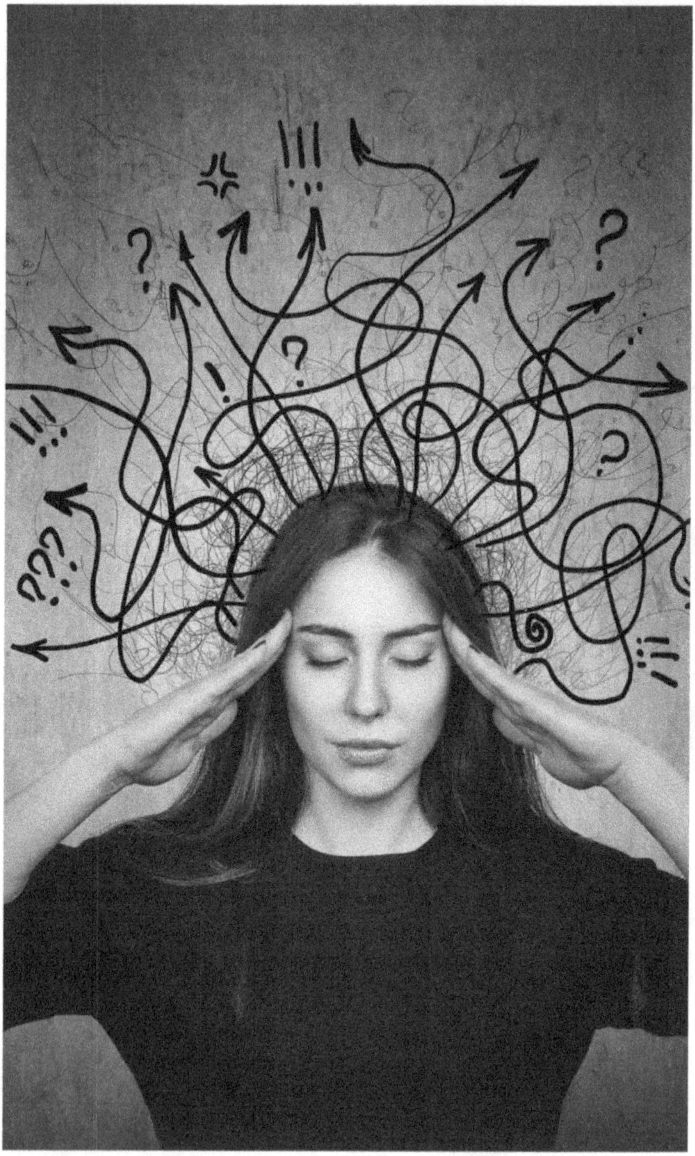

INTRODUCTION

Overthinking and stress have a method for fusing itself into any part of a women's life. Regardless of whether it comes as a total frenzy or a consistent concern, overthinking or stress can confine any piece of your life's latent capacity. It could keep you from going to class, prevent you from getting a new line of work, devastate your fellowships or even render you a detainee in your home. To put it plainly, it tends to be totally impairing.

Living with extreme overthinking/anxiety or concern will cause it hard to feel inspired to find support. This is particularly obvious on the off chance that you have been taking drugs and have not seen any improvement. Down to earth, simple to-follow approaches are required to offer you a direct guide towards progress.

Here is the place this book comes in. Every day, women suffer from overthinking behaviors that can lead to them feeling an increase in stress, nervousness, unworthiness, being overwhelmed, and obligation to those around them. Overthinking naturally stems from a desire to attempt to control every possible outcome of a situation, but unfortunately, it only results in the absolute certainty that the woman engaging in it will feel more stressed and overwhelmed than ever before.

The book will show you the methods you can use to manage and stop overthinking, rather than instructing you.

Can utilizing thoughts from a self-improvement guide about brain research help diminish superfluous nerves and fears? Answer is yes. Quit overthinking and stress incorporates loads of thoughts, indications, and exercises to assist you with handling your issue. You'll better see how to conquer overthinking practices in this book, and increment your odds of wellbeing and joy. You can gain genuine ground against the feelings of thought which frequent you by teaching yourself and executing what you know.

This book contains direction on the most proficient method to deal with your feelings of trepidation and stress, showing that there is a lot to know and do. The advantageous style of the exercise manual empowers you to take this information in and use it at your own speed. It is important to work at your own pace, since it ordinarily sets aside some effort to process new thoughts, pick activities, and plan your reactions to fear, check your arrangement, and make updates focused on what you have realized.

Stop overthinking and stress is a stage. It's something that occurs after some time, where you are causing changes as you to go. You increase far reaching authority of the procedures through this stage which will assist you with limiting or resolve unnecessary apprehensions.

You will conclude how to cause pace for yourself so you can feel positive about the possibilities instead of feeling overpowered by all the potential choices. Loosen up a little to perceive what you can do.

My fundamental interest from you is that you devote yourself to overseeing this book as far as possible. This book is for those that are overthinking—regardless of whether you're as of now experiencing guiding, dithering to start, or not yet having the devices to look for outside help. In spite of the fact that the point of this book isn't to substitute an advisor, the methods talked about here are a similar that you would learn in treatment. Make this book your accomplice in obligation in a quest for good psychological well-being and freedom from stress. You've finished the principal significant move to begin reading this book. We should proceed.

CHAPTER ONE: UNDERSTANDING OVERTHINKING AND STRESS

In this part, we'll talk about overthinking and stress, recognize its different structures, and recommend treatment styles for it. Eventually, you'll get a comprehension of the sort of stress and overthinking you're feeling, how it creates in your body and psyche, and why it's important to act to oversee it.

1.1. The Anxious Mind and Body

The Mental Disorders Diagnostic and Statistical Manual depict stress as the "desire for future damage." Those with overthinking feel pressure, worried about potential dangers, and oppose possibly risky conditions.

OVERTHINKING IN THE BRAIN

An attack of nervousness begins with the tangible receptors: ears, eyes, nose. Simply envision Sarah tuning in to the doorbell. In her mind stem neurons are starting to more liberate all the more unequivocally. Synapses like norepinephrine offers data to parts of her mind and yell, "Cautioning, cautioning!"

ANXIETY IN THE BODY

Think about a circumstance where you've experienced overthinking — review how you reacted? Did you feel befuddled or apprehensive by it? Have you had physical side effects like shaking, or a heartbeat hustling?

1.2. The Source of Overthinking and stress

A few people experience on edge sentiments for their entire lives; others experience overthinking simply after an episode or injury has caused it. Overthinking is thought to emerge from a blend of components separating for every individual. Hereditary qualities, which are parts of your beginning periods of improvement, are expected to have an impact.

Any individuals from the family at any point had nervousness analyzed? Twin discoveries are utilized to assess the job of hereditary qualities in scatters of stress since indistinguishable twins have similar qualities. An audit of twin discoveries found in the American Journal of Psychiatry in 2001 said hereditary qualities contributed 30 to 40 percent to the wellspring of nervousness issue. This infers stress for the most part runs in families and on the off chance that somebody in your family as of now has one you are progressively inclined to building up an overthinking issue.

It is additionally accepted that ecological elements assume a significant job in overthinking. Occasions, for example, savagery or an excessively basic parent may cause stress during youth.

Occasions in life that the vast majority experience can cause nervousness in the individuals who are as of now in danger because of their hereditary components, for example, movement, relationship issues, and loss of friends and family. Seeing an on-edge parent can likewise make you bound to procure a nervousness issue yourself, since you gain from your parent's knowledge and begin to build up a similar personal behavioral standard.

Explicit fears, similar to the fear of tallness, consistently have a quick beginning: a situation that hasn't caused you overthinking or inconvenience before abruptly turns into a wellspring of stress. For this situation, the reason could be a sharpening event like terrible disturbance on a battle. At the point when you are adapted to overthinking, your psyche can think that it’s hard to relinquish the occasion's memory, and wind up making you be careful about a similar future danger.

Have you taken nervousness prescription? Assuming this is the case, what was your opinion about it? Have you discovered that your side effects improved, and has the improvement gone on as long as possible? In the event that you had never taken medicine for stress, okay discover it?

1.3. Anxiety

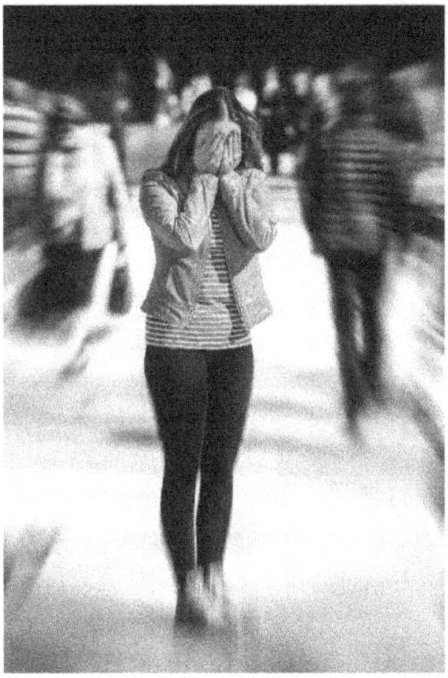

Anxiety is definitely not a single direction issue; it very well may be introduced in a few different ways. Five types of anxiety issue are set out underneath. In every particular example, a stress issue is possibly given a finding when fear causes huge life impedance and has been dynamic for a long time.

EXCEPTIONAL PHOBIA

People with one of kind fears are alarmed of things or conditions like creatures or statures. Numerous fears are about things a great many people thought; be that as it may, in those with nervousness, the thought or stress is out of examination with the real peril. An individual who fears pooches may discover visiting companions who own mutts troublesome. Someone with a fear of needles may forestall looking for huge clinical consideration. One of a kind fears are presented when an individual's life is seriously influenced by stress over a time of months.

OPEN ANXIETY DISORDER

Individuals with open overthinking issue (PAD) have a staggering apprehension that they will be embarrassed or censured in social or execution conditions, for example, setting off to a gathering or talking. They might be hesitant to grin, shake or act in manners that will make individuals believe they're peculiar or anxious.

FRENZY DISORDER

Frenzy issue causes extreme, abrupt fits of anxiety with crippling side effects, for example, a quick heartbeat, trouble breathing, chest agony and queasiness. The individual ought to relate them to a clinical reason when these assaults happen first, and visit the emergency clinic looking for help. People with alarm issue may feel insane, and might be stressed over more assaults.

AGORAPHOBIA

People with agoraphobia are hesitant to be in places where it would be practically difficult to get away or get help in the event that they had a fit of anxiety, as in a jam-packed cinema. In these conditions they may think: "Imagine a scenario in which I alarm and can't simply leave, what will occur?" Some people with agoraphobia feel great with a believed companion or family while others evade totally venturing out from home. A great many people encountering agoraphobia have gone through a half year or additionally managing their nervousness.

THE GENERALIZED ANXIETY DISORDER (GAD)

The summed-up nervousness issue incorporates serious, diligent concern. Those with GAD are concerned with wellbeing, funds, relatives, encountering a mishap—about all. On the off chance that one concern leaves, it has its spot to another. These feelings of trepidation proceed for a long time and are frequently trailed by physical manifestations. Showing signs of improvement.

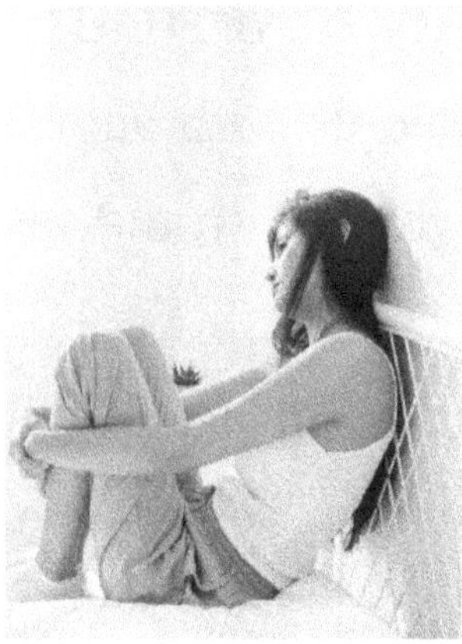

It very well may be overpowering to attempt intellectual behavioral treatment or different treatments just because, particularly when you believe you have done everything and nothing has been powerful. Unfurling nervousness may feel like you are being exposed to more torment. However, some way or another the outcome is justified, despite all the trouble.

Here is a rundown of ways that overcoming nervousness that will change your life:

- It's going to make your life objectives simpler to achieve. You would don't hesitate to pursue that advancement or take that long-venture trip when you are not any more apprehensive and maintaining a strategic distance from conditions. Objectives that showed up far off may out of nowhere work out as expected.

- You will take a gander at your future in an increasingly idealistic manner. Overthinking tends to cast a negative point of view toward something that is yet to come. At the point when you're effortless, you'll feel progressively idealistic about what might be on the horizon.
- Medical issues will be made simpler to manage. You're not going to be stressed over your physical wellbeing unnecessarily, yet rather will do what's expected to take legitimate consideration of yourself. Specialist visits won't fill you with overthinking and stress any more.
- You would feel assuaged from low state of mind or sadness. Wretchedness and low state of mind frequently exhibit change as nervousness is diminished.
- As well as feeling less discouraged, you can feel increasingly certain, have additional time, rest

better and have more enthusiasm for life when all is said in done.

- Anxiety doesn't depict you as a human any more. On the off chance that you have extensive held convictions of yourself that is based around being on edge, sentiments of confidence and self-esteem would supplant them. Without those on edge musings you'll get the chance to comprehend the individual you can be.
- You'll be dealing with yourself better. Conquering trepidation will sparkle a light on the neglected aspects of your life. You'll put more accentuation on things like exercise, nourishment, and being available right now.
- It will fortify kinships and ventures that have endured. You may grow new social bonds, or you may feel less dependent on individuals you have recently depended on. Your improved capacity to focus will make the undertakings resemble an errand, and you may even end up searching for work environment progression.

You'll encounter improved deep-rooted joy and more certainty. Overthinking and stress has an approach to destroy your delight and certainty. In the event that you have felt like you are simply "traversing" each day, you're going to start every day excitedly and looking for delight.

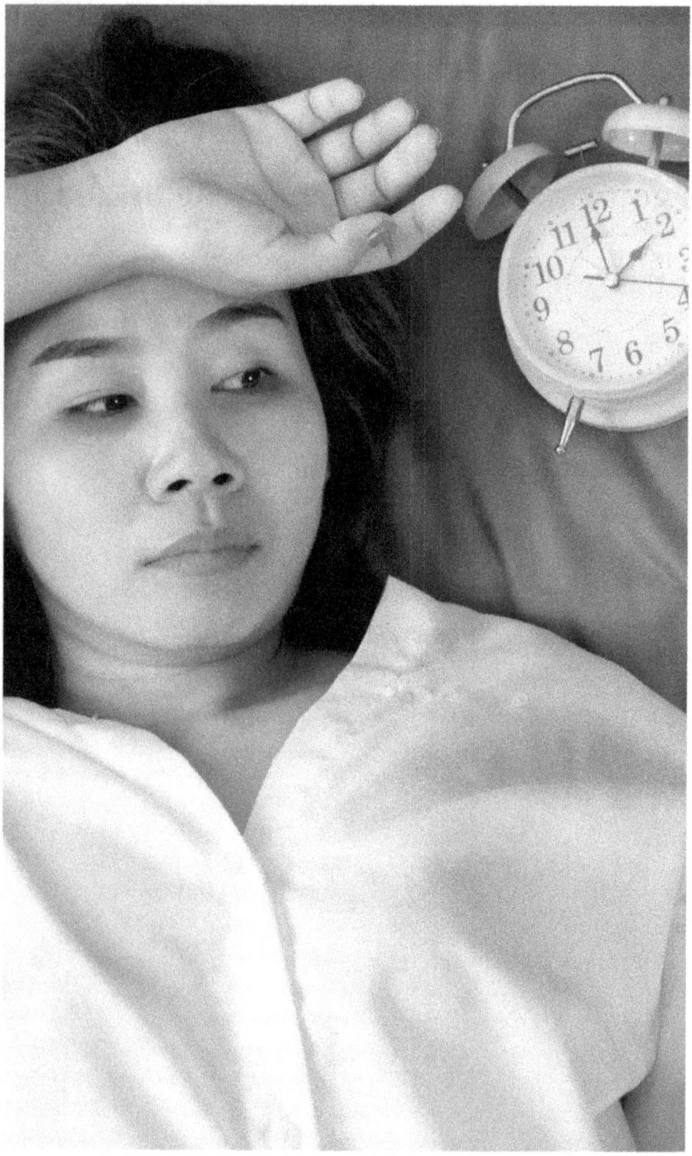

CHAPTER TWO: THE COGNITIVE BEHAVIORAL APPROACH TO STOP OVERTHINKING AND STRESS

We'll find out about Cognitive behavioral treatment in this part, including how the procedure started, its center ideas and why it works. In the wake of perusing this part you ought to see better how CBT can help with your stress.

INTELLECTUAL BEHAVIORAL THERAPY: A BRIEF HISTORY

The sources of CBT go back to the Ancient Greece Times. The Greek rationalist Epictetus, for instance, who confronted significant difficulties on his own method to progress, guaranteed that thinking could be utilized to perceive and dismiss deceptions prompting damaging feelings. In any case, cognitive social treatment didn't get main stream until the 1980s.

EARLY BEGINNINGS

They guarantee need is the mother of advancement and it was the same as the most punctual phases of CBT. A surge of World War II veterans experienced nervousness and sorrow by the late 1940s and clinicians were scanning for transient medicines. Freudian psychoanalytic treatment, which around then was the most mainstream treatment, no longer addressed the issues of patients or advisors. At the skirt of progress was the mental analysis.

You have found out about the Russian physiologist Ivan Pavlov, most likely. It was during the 1890s that he set up the adapted reflex idea. He uncovered in his examination that hounds that had been taken care of at a ringer's tone unexpectedly started to salivate when the chime rang. Pavlov's exploration has been instrumental in exhibiting how thought could be molded. At that point, in 1920, Pavlov's work was extended by the American formative therapist John B. Watson. In the trial called "Little Albert" he demonstrated that when joined with an uproarious clamor, a small kid could figure out how to fear fuzzy animals. Thereafter American analyst B. F. Skinner, with his guideline of operant molding, showed how motivating force and discipline could impact behavioral. Another medication dependent on these thoughts, called behavioral treatment, was progressively evolved in a few regions of the world by the 1950s and 1960s. Early remedial methodologies concentrated on expanding affectability to fear boosts or conditions like deliberate desensitization established by specialist Joseph Wolpe from South Africa. Behavioral mediations stay a basic component of CBT right up 'til today.

SECOND WAVE

By the late 1960s, the mental field had been prepared for additional change. The essentialness of musings (comprehensions) had been perceived in feelings and behavioral, and the intellectual unrest began to come to fruition. In the reasonable transformation, clinicians were presently thinking about the feelings of patients instead of simply their behavioral. Rather than considering people to be Pavlov's canines, promptly reacting to an outside occasion, it was comprehended that contemplations were the association between outer occasions and feelings and practices.

Along these lines, CBT looked for not exclusively to adjust behavioral, yet in addition convictions, mentalities, methods for thought and desires. The psychological and behavioral strategies converged during the 1980s and 1990s to frame this new sort of treatment.

Compelling figures during this period included American clinician Albert Ellis, the maker of Rational Emotional Behavior Therapy (REBT) and American specialist Aaron T. Beck, the pioneer of cognitive treatment.

THIRD WAVE

CBT by and by transformed with the new thousand years. During what is viewed as the third wave, when arranging treatment, advisors respected the way toward thinking itself, instead of just the substance of the musings. On the off chance that I requested that you cease from pondering chocolate cake at the present time, what is the primary thing that comes into view? Eating obviously, a wanton cut. As indicated by this ongoing flood of CBT it was worthless to attempt to control contemplations and feelings. During this period, new treatments like acknowledgment and commitment treatment (ACT) and persuasive social treatment (DBT) rose which incorporated the job of acknowledgment and consideration into ordinary CBT.

CBT has become the standard type of treatment for an assortment of mental issue, paying little mind to the fundamental procedures utilized. We will talk about the CBT strategy in the following section, and why it works.

2.1. Why and How

CBT's center standards can be separated into two fundamental topics: useful cooperation and formal critical thinking. At the point when we examine various parts of CBT you will find that the attention is on time sensitive treatment. Due to the normalized idea of this program, most customers will end their consideration inside weeks to a couple of months.

SUCCESSFUL COLLABORATION

Cooperating

Envision participating in treatment with a specialist who can give talks and depreciate you. Regardless of whether the medicines were successful, you would no longer feel in charge of your own adapting abilities. In correlation, the advisor and customer cooperate on a quest for development during CBT. This methodology depends on a solid shared collusion; CBT advisors are empathic, mindful, acceptable audience members, strong of your accomplishments and request contribution from you. We portray how considerations and practices, through a procedure called controlled learning, lead to stress. This incorporates investigating realities, testing for legitimacy of thoughts, revealing oblivious considerations, and producing more reactions—together.

In view of training

CBT customers are not just practicing new aptitudes. We likewise catch wind of their stress issue and the CBT approach that underlies them. Instruction is a huge part of such treatment.

Powerful and expertise situated

The therapist and customer examine together during CBT on what to deal with, how and when to meet and what to accomplish for assignments. With time, the customer assumes a progressively dynamic job and creates procedures to forestall backslide once the treatment is finished.

Features practicality

Consistently you can't turn off your cerebrum for a second, and let another person fix you in CBT. To pick up from this type of treatment you need to do the exploration.

You should concentrate on the current stage

Rather than harping on the wellsprings of your trouble, CBT intends to get it down in the present. The past is possibly intriguing to consider on the off chance that it leaves you caught with your issues.

Restricted time

In 6 to 20 meetings most clients with slight to direct issues can be upheld. Promoter meetings are likewise frequently utilized toward the finish of the treatment to fortify what you have realized; however, CBT is a time sensitive treatment.

Developed

Each CBT procedure follows a normalized design: registration, investigation of the earlier week, motivation of the present week, survey of the schoolwork, issues of the present week, setting up new schoolwork, summarizing and accepting input. Thusly, after determination, customers realize what to foresee and can utilize similar norms themselves.

In view of proof

CBT utilizes a scope of systems that have been tried and appeared to work. The specialist utilizes CBT approaches that are known to work better for the difficulties a specific customer face.

2.2. Inspiration for progress

A few people battle with a stress related inspiration for progress. Maybe the hindrances appear to be too enormous regularly, when arranging a change, people experience five phases:

- Pre-consideration: in the pre-thought stage, you figure your nervousness can be limited yet you have not yet committed to rolling out an improvement.

- Consideration: At the purpose of thought, you hope to work at some point later on diminishing your overthinking however have not yet made any move to do as such.
- Readiness: You are effectively arranging how to ease your stress in the short term during the planning time frame.
- Activity: You are intentionally taking a shot at making a move regarding your stress through the activity stage.
- Upkeep: You're working in the support procedure not to slip once again into old propensities for apprehensive reasoning and practices.

You've just experienced the initial two stages in case you understand this and effectively want to fix your stress and overthinking. In the event that you are as yet unfit to focus on progress, ask yourself the key inquiries:

What are the upsides/drawbacks of the overthinking treatment? What's more, on the off chance that you despite everything have thought and overthinking, by what method will your life look like quite a while from now?

How could that be going to look on the off chance that you don't?

2.3. Promise to prosperity

While I've attempted to cause this book as direct as I to can, it's despite everything up to you to carry out the responsibility. Life is probably going to send you some curves throughout the following barely any weeks—kindly don't let this stop you. Much the same as you endeavor to set aside a few minutes for work out, rest soundly and get enough rest, set aside a few minutes for this.

Your mental wellbeing needs the same amount of consideration.

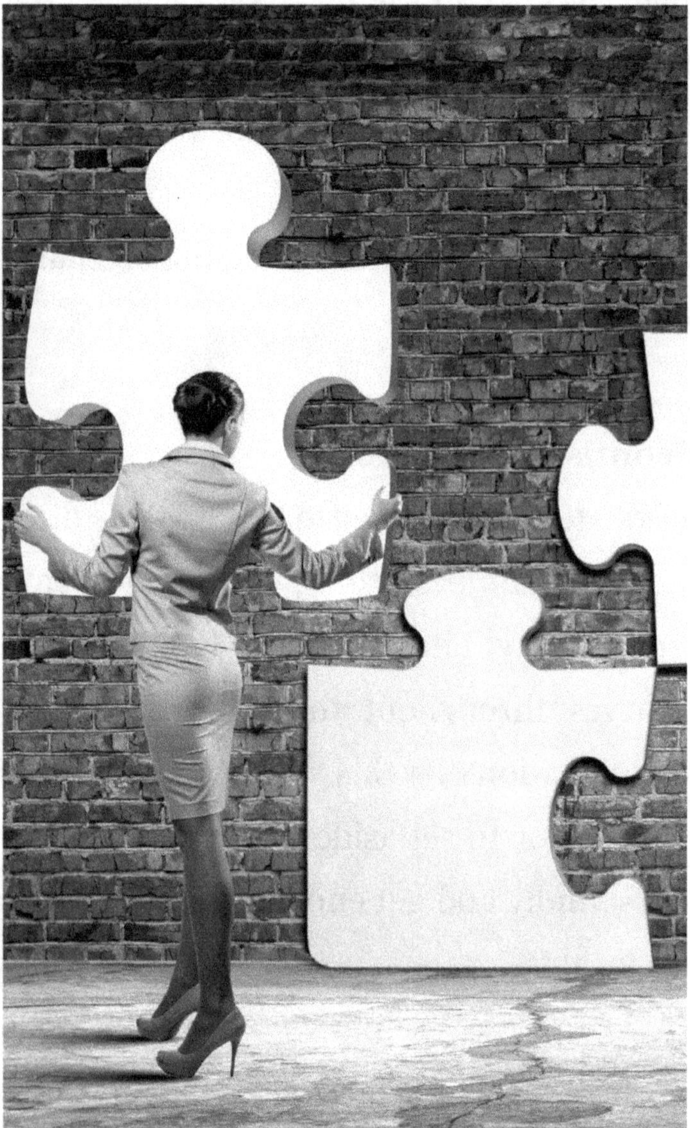

CHAPTER THREE: WHAT TROUBLES YOU?

I caught wind of the subjective social way to deal with overseeing overthinking in the past part in regard to the setting of CBT and why it works. We have spoken about the drive to improve and to adhere to wellbeing.

Before we start on CBT's specialized perspectives, it's imperative to consider the goals that you're wanting to accomplish by following up on your nervousness. To set objectives, we will initially break down stress and specific signs in your center issues. Everyone has a particular arrangement of issues—even two individuals determined to have a similar stress and overthinking.

3.1. Understanding the Downturn

Which overthinking side effects do you stress generally over? Which parts of your life were generally influenced by your concerns? Distinguishing your specific side effects and the spots where help is required is a key advance in defining objectives.

Bring one moment to record your musings. Are there certain pieces of your life you feel like required consideration regarding? Which kinds of side effects of stress make life much harder for you? Think about an ongoing occasion in which you have felt anxiety and record portions of the circumstance in your brain that stick out.

PHYSICAL SIDE EFFECTS

Recollect your most present stress experience. What were your sentiments? While examining the various sorts of stress issue, we tended to a portion of these indications. Check the most extreme side effects for you, which cause the most agony in your regular day to day existence.

- Blurred vision
- Lips trembling
- Chest torment
- Weeping
- Selecting sensation
- Lightheadedness or dazedness

- Dry mouth
- Heavy perspiring
- Exhaustion
- Feelings of vacancy or confinement
- Cerebral pains
- Body solidness
- Nausea or looseness of the bowels
- Numbness or shivering
- Pounding or shivering heart
- Shaky discourse
- Breathlessness or covering sensation
- Trembling or shaking
- Discomfort arm
- Others...

MENTAL SIDE EFFECTS

Mental side effects imply your overthinking enthusiastic encounters. Such manifestations vary as per the particular nervousness type. At the point when you're getting a frenzy issue, you're concerned you will go crazy. In the event that you have a social nervousness issue, you thought that you are being seen in a contrary way by others.

Consider your new disturbing experience.
- Considerations experienced your brain? For what reason did the overthinking influence your mind-set or focus?

Check the manifestations underneath that allude to you, and note any side effects not secured.

- I was frightened that others were making a decision about me.
- I was frightened to be humiliated or disregarded.
- I anticipated that a social or achievement occasion should come.
- I felt like things were going to end gravely.
- I felt anxious and keyed up.
- I was terrified to lose control or go frantic.
- I was reluctant to be dead.

- I was anxious about the possibility that that on the off chance that I got terrified; I couldn't generally break free.
- I had the impending sentiment of calamity.
- I had an inclination that I expected to run.
- I battled to center.
- My heart went dry.
- I was feeling crabby.
- I lost classification.
- I was unable to adapt.
- I felt totally miserable.
- I had a feeling that I had no power over my concerns.
- Other...

SOCIAL SIDE EFFECTS

Overthinking doesn't show alone in what you feel or what you look like it's reflected in your behavioral as well. On the off chance that you have a frenzy issue, in light of the thought of having a fit of anxiety and not having the option to get away, you may abstain from taking lifts. In the event that you have a snake fear, you may conclude occasions to tropical retreats are impossible. Social stress can prompt you staying away from parties or other social duties. The following are a few manners by which stress can show itself in your behavioral. Allude to the circumstance you portrayed toward the start of this area, check the examples underneath that are legitimate for you, and record in any that isn't recorded.

- I evaded the things I feared, or conditions.
- I've overcompensated by the extra difficult work.
- I fled the circumstance, or got away.
- I have gotten things done to loosen up myself or not feel anxious (e.g., I don't see somebody in the eye).
- I was looking for consolation from individuals somewhere else.

3.2. Behavioral Approach Test

Advisors/Professionals frequently utilize a device called the social methodology test (BAT) to make physical, mental, and behavioral indications of stress simpler to distinguish. You should arrive at a feared situation utilizing this strategy and afterward quickly a while later make notes of your nervousness side effects and practices.

In certain circumstances, it may be too apprehensive to possibly be confronted with a thought circumstance.

At the point when you experience issues perceiving the indications of nervousness, look for your very own investigation helpful methodology. Join a condition that you thought, and afterward report your anxious sentiments, contemplations, and practices promptly a short time later. In the event that that sounds excessively overpowering, do a pretend wherein you feel that you are entering the condition. Pen down any inquiries you have with respect to this activity.

3.3. Nervousness Inception

Fathoming your overthinking triggers—those conditions that add to your stress experience—is an essential piece of recuperation arranging. While a portion of your stress may appear to be free-coasting and not related with a particular reason, a portion of your side effects may show up typically.

The overthinking manifestations are commonly simple to distinguish on account of genuine fears. In case you're anxious about statures, you'll feel stressed over a structure on a high floor. In case you're anxious about needles, when hanging tight for an influenza shot, you'll feel the thought rising.

The reasons for social nervousness issue spread an assortment of social and execution conditions. Some nervousness inciting situations incorporate conversing with outsiders, meeting another person, asking somebody out on the town, imparting your insight or setting off to a request for employment. Regular commencements for execution remember drinking or eating for front of everybody, writing before others, addressing the group and utilizing an open can.

The reasons for overthinking in the occurrence of frenzy issue incorporate body boosts and the view of them. On the off chance that you have alarm issue, you are commonly receptive to your body's feelings and see them in an overwhelming way. Chest torment is known as a coronary failure. Getting trouble holding your breath is hyperventilation. For alarm issue, stress that your manifestations are a sign of a hidden medical issue is a typical trigger.

In the event that you have agoraphobia, your thought is most likely activated by conditions that you feel it is difficult to get away on the off chance that you had a fit of anxiety, such as driving on open vehicle, being in open or shut spaces, remaining in groups or lines, and being distant from everyone else out of your home. What conditions or things would you say you fear, or maintain a strategic distance from? What components of specific things or conditions escalate your stress? Recall when you first feel truly stressed, or had a fit of anxiety? Consider about what was happening at that point, and a particular part of the case.

3.4. Center zones

We have been gabbing about the particular side effects of nervousness. I might likewise want to find out about various aspects of your life, and how they add to your overthinking. The personal satisfaction is regularly decreased because of stress. Educational encounters can likewise now and again cause or strengthen nervousness, for example, working in a requesting work or getting a separation. Your present condition of life is the sense wherein your stress has continued, so it is essential that we get it.

We should pause for a moment to analyze each part of your life now. I'd like you to concentrate on how you're doing, how you realize you need change, and how you have nervousness.

SOCIAL ENCOUNTERS

Nervousness can prompt issues in your connections and relationship issues will exacerbate your stress also. Social overthinking can make you feel confined.

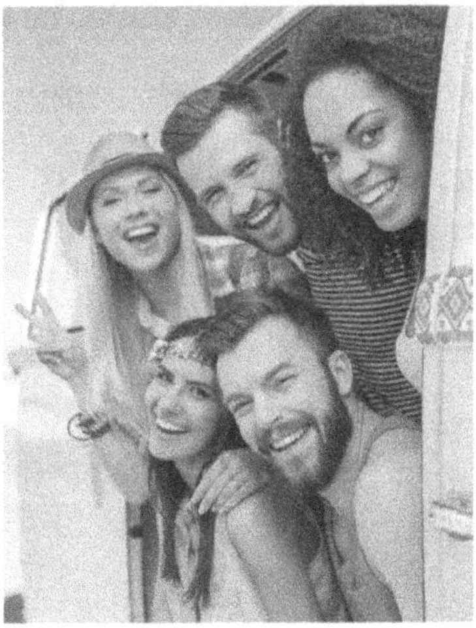

This makes it hard to produce new associations. Fits of anxiety could leave you embarrassed. The shame of having nervousness can regularly act like a lot of a weight as the indications of overthinking itself.

What's more, issues with connections can prompt overthinking. Upsetting conditions like a separation can create new worries that add to the pressure and make it hard to adapt.

Think about your own one-of-a-kind character. How did the thought influence your connections? You may consider your family members, companions, sentimental accomplice or children, contingent upon whose present in your life. Do you have a Partner? Did you face any adjustments in your connections? Is it true that you are battling to frame new companions? Compose back your sentiments.

TRAINING AND WORK

In what ways did nervousness affect your instruction or vocation? Would it be a good idea for you to continually stress over the duty regarding the work? Did you drop out of school or go home out of thought of leaving the house? Have you abstained from taking exercises or working at a vocation where it takes open talking? Does pressure add to your stress at work? Consider how your instruction or employment has impacted the stress. What is your opinion about your current circumstance at school or at work? Compose your appearance.

WELLBEING

Stress will antagonistically influence your wellbeing and prosperity. This can meddle with your capacity to keep up your own wellbeing, for example, keeping up a solid eating routine or day by day work out. Medical issues can likewise compound nervousness issues, for example, alarm activating asthma assaults.

In like manner, headaches and touchy gut disorder will in general oblige nervousness and can make torment you. You may even have psychological wellness issues that cover, for example, despondency or substance misuse, which can make it a lot harder to vanquish stress.

We should consider your general wellbeing and prosperity for a second. Did you get any ailments or other psychological well-being conditions that could prompt your overthinking? How are you resting? It is safe to say that you are eating well nourishments? Accomplish you turn out consistently? Stress can influence incredible entirety regions, and they can likewise influence your nervousness, so it's critical to recollect how you're doing.

ORDINARY DUTIES

This classification incorporates things that you generally do each day, for example, driving a vehicle, making suppers, dealing with yourself, taking care of tabs, cleaning the house, picking garments to wear, and so on. Stress can debilitate your capacity to play out the least complex undertakings. How is your capacity to fulfill each day's needs? Was thought playing with completing things? Are your days so insane and distressing, that your overthinking deteriorates? Pen your emotions.

DIFFERENT VARIABLES

Are there some other aspects of your life that we haven't addressed, for example, your money related circumstance, lodging issues, security and wellbeing considerations, or relaxation time? Recall how these could add to your stress, and record your considerations underneath.

Did you face any ongoing money related difficulties, for instance? It is safe to say that you are not loosened up where you live? Do you have any motivation to feel risky around you? Do you possess energy for rest and fun, and would you be able to appreciate it? Compose your appearance.

3.5. Objective Setting

Is it true that you are prepared to set your objectives? I for one am energized that we are in the process at this stage. It is here that we start to find a way to assist you with defeating your overthinking. Objectives are essential to the procedure as they let you check whether you've gained any ground. These can incorporate momentary gains or long haul alterations, and might be of a general sort or spotlight on a particular worry by laser.

Momentary objectives are the ones you may achieve inside the following week, medium-go objectives that take two or three weeks, and long-run objectives are the ones you hope to reach inside the following year or two.

Objectives can be general or interesting, as well. Clear objectives are useful when arranging undertakings during treatment, though by and large objectives consider the wide picture of what you are attempting to achieve through treatment.

For instance, Jane has picked the accompanying generally speaking objectives with a medium time span (by treatment finishing):

1. Think less on edge and stressed over her regular daily existence.
2. Work hours more attractive.
3. Improve her connection with her significant other.
4. It expands her confidence in herself.
5. Feel certain about her physical wellbeing.

In light of these general destinations, she grew clear momentary objectives in care, for example, working no longer than 40 hours out of every week and practicing three days per week for 35 minutes.

OBJECTIVES SET

It's your turn now. Glancing back at what we have shrouded in this section, including the physical, mental, and social side effects, and their consequences for different everyday issues. Considering the key topics that emerge, think of four to six general objectives that you would like to achieve by the consummation of this program. Compose these down. Try not to freeze about explicit targets coming up as of now—we'll discover those in a later part.

3.6. The Stress Journal

A Stress Journal is a valuable apparatus to track how frequently you experience nervousness causing conditions, what you feel in those conditions, how you react and the degree of your misery.

Each time you experience huge overthinking, note the date and time, condition, rating your thought or stress from 0 to 10, and any physical sentiments you have felt, feelings you have had and moves you have made. Note, behavioral can in some cases incorporate evasion, for example, escaping a circumstance. Give filling a shot the structure not long after the occasion, so you can rapidly recall what occurred. Want to finish this structure whenever you go over a stressed circumstance throughout the following week.

3.7. Tending to Uncertainty

Do you feel questionable whether CBT can work or marvel if it's proper for you? On the off chance that this is along these lines, we should discuss your concerns for a second. CBT has been demonstrated to be useful in stress recuperation; however it takes devotion on your part. In the event that you were in overthinking treatment previously, or try an ineffectual self-improvement plan, you might be asking why this time will be any unique. How about we take one moment to take a gander at your stress prescription history.

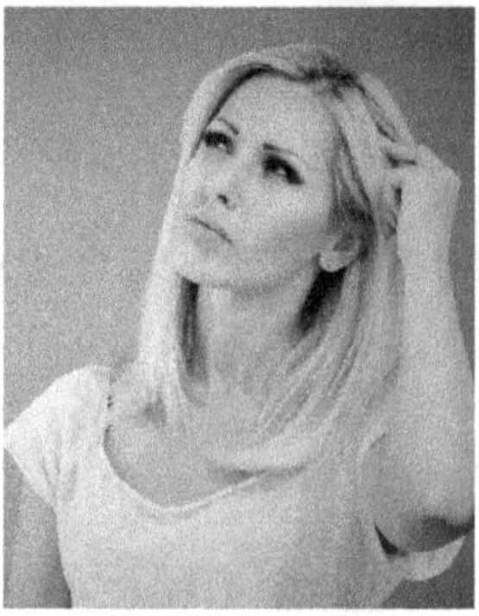

Report some other types of advising you have, and any self-improvement guides you utilized previously. Portray to what extent everything endured and on the off chance that you saw any changes. In the event that they weren't canning, you think about any causes why? Did you feel regarded in that relationship, on the off chance that you saw an advisor? In the event that you utilized a book of self-improvement, have you tried the thoughts? How about we adopt your impression of the strategy to CBT now. What's your opinion about CBT when all is said in done up till now? Okay need to invest energy consistently to give these qualities something to do? Do you think this procedure bodes well and can work for you? Make notes about your CBT desires and what you want to accomplish by following the exercises in this book here.

YOUR QUALITIES

At the point when you're on edge, it is anything but difficult to be centered on your issues. At the point when you're canvassed in what you've fouled up, what you will foul up, and what may turn out badly, your qualities make some hard memories coming up to the surface. Be that as it may, every individual has various qualities which can assist with settling even the most exceedingly terrible circumstances. For Jane's situation, her work was foremost; when her stress has been leveled out, advancement was probably going to be given.

At the point when you've managed overthinking for quite a while, contemplating yourself about positive stuff may be hard. To help you with this crucial, of these. What are you splendid at? You may consistently focus on detail or you might be a characteristic coordinator. Did you conquer any critical life deterrents, for example, figuring out how to adapt to a clinical issue? How could you help or satisfy others, possibly by being a decent audience or offering guidance? Have you any special characteristics, similar to an idiosyncratic comical inclination? At last, what are you most esteeming for? I appreciate time went through with my family for instance, voyaging and discovering some new information. Record your contemplations. Through that procedure, expanding on your qualities will be advantageous.

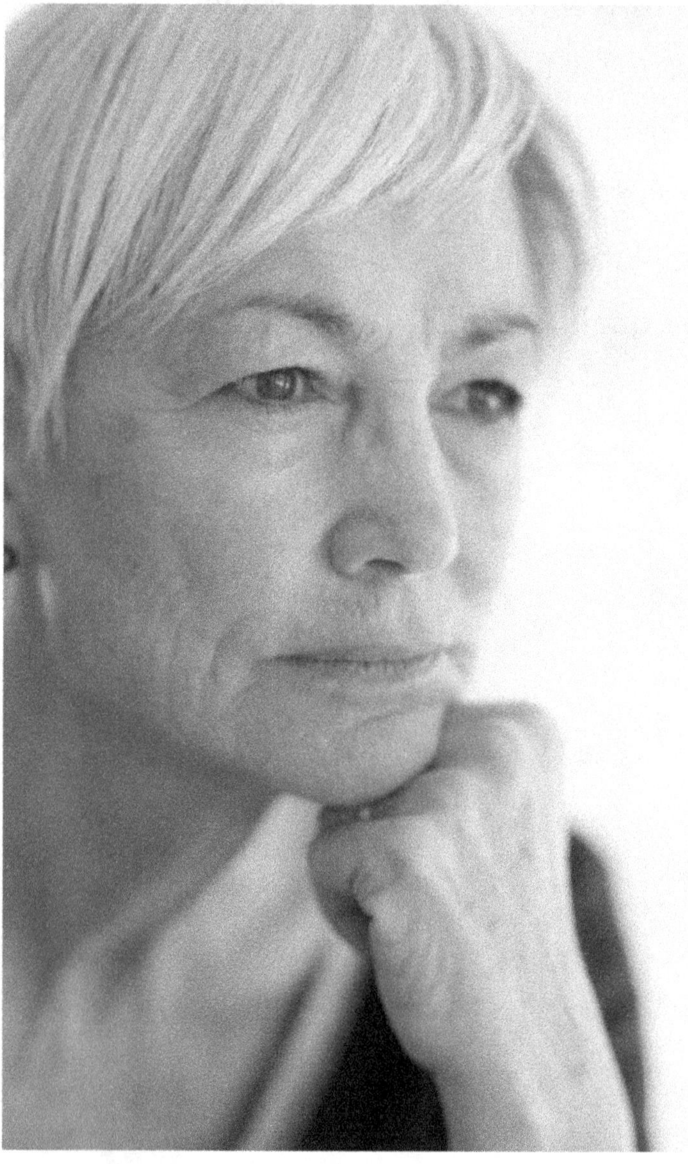

CHAPTER FOUR: FIND THE PATTERNS OF YOUR THOUGHT

We examined the manifestations of overthinking in the last part, and how various pieces of your life add to your nervousness. Thus, we set some broad targets that you will try to accomplish by the finishing of this program. I additionally requested that you keep an overthinking Journal where you revealed conditions that made you stressed—you wrote down what you felt, thought, and did at every one of those occasions.

How did your Stress Journal turn out? Experience you experienced issues making sense of how you felt, or what you thought? Try not to burn through an excessive amount of time on this—in the second piece of this portion we'll burrow further to perceive the musings that separate conditions and your apprehensive responses.

In the first place, I'd prefer to begin by talking about the different ways considerations can be unhelpful when you're on edge.

4.1. Overthinking Considerations Types

On edge musings for the most part follow predictable examples. Among these patterns, the most mainstream are those that anticipate something negative occurring later on, those that incorporate self-analysis, and those that speak to a feeling of edginess. How about we take a gander at of all of these sorts of on edge contemplations

WHAT IF?

The greater part of our restless contemplations comes as remarks like 'imagine a scenario in which.' "Consider the possibility that I got assaulted by that hound?" "Consider the possibility that my treatment doesn't work?" "Imagine a scenario where when I'm at supper and my hands begin shaking?" "Imagine a scenario where I'm in that lift and I experience a fit of anxiety?" These announcements, as should be obvious, by and large incorporate hopping to a supposition about what could happen later on and foreseeing the most exceedingly terrible would occur. We call that "calamitous," or the demonstration of screwing things messed up.

Such type of concern may likewise include guessing what you might be thinking or accepting you comprehends what others are thinking. This is especially evident on account of social nervousness issue. You're most likely reasoning a great deal — about terrible things that may occur later on, and how individuals will react to them.

You could likewise reach determinations about what your body's sentiments mean.

This last proclamation is particularly evident in the event that you have a frenzy issue — you likely accept on the off chance that you feel restless it must imply that there is something to be stressed over.

In any case, sentiments can have a great deal of triggers and don't generally reflect reality. Do you have a ton of musings on "consider the possibility that? Record a not many that you think about recognizable to you.

THE PUNDIT

Stress can drive you to considerations that incorporate analysis or a craving for flawlessness. You dissect conditions that occurred; focus just on what turned out badly and overlook such went right.

Considerations along these terms ordinarily go like "That was moronic," or "I must do everything right." You consider it to be highly contrasting, valid or bogus, right or wrong. In the event that you spill refreshment at a gathering, that implies you've destroyed the entire occasion, messed everything up, and you're never going to be welcomed back again. Personalization joins compulsiveness—accusing yourself for characteristic occasions beyond your ability to do anything about. At the point when you have a typical overthinking issue, you are potentially experiencing issues adapting to disarray and may trust you need to do whatever you can to guarantee victory. In the case of something awful occurs, you're feeling mindful—like you could have gone somewhat further to keep away from it.

What kind of basic reasoning do you have concerning yourself? Recognize, and record a portion of these.

ACTING THE PERSON IN QUESTION

At the point when you battle with overthinking, you may have sentiments about not having the option to accomplish something. Your assessments will come the lines of "I can't work with others who don't care for me," or "I can't disregard the house, I can't deal with it on the off chance that I begin to freeze." This regularly comes as overgeneralization—making one occasion a more concerning issue. You may think, "In case I'm behind schedule for work, I will fizzle at my particular employment." As another model, a terrible involvement in a canine would mean you should fear all pooches.

Overgeneralization can include giving you names, as well. Inferable from your social cumbersomeness, you could call yourself "odd," "unusual," or "exhausting," while at the same time overlooking the entirety of your positive attributes.

Which thoughts do you have that propose an inclination that you can't adapt? Record a portion of these.

4.2. Distinguishing your thoughts

Think about an ongoing circumstance in which you felt restless about yourself. You may have discovered one in your Overthinking Journal which can be utilized for instance here. What occasion have you gotten? Just consider it clearly as you can.

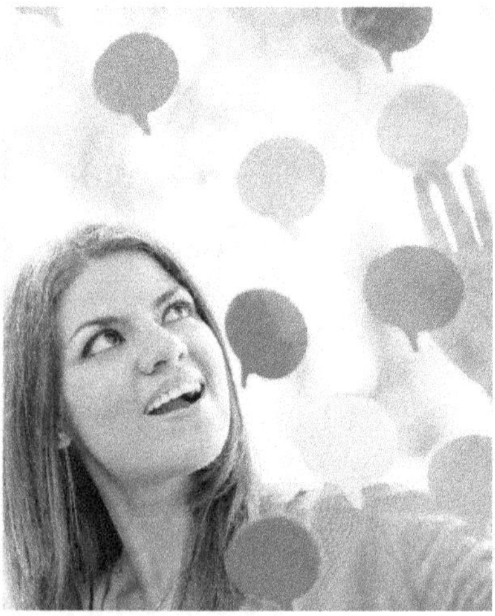

Where you, who was there and what were was the hour of day? Occasions can be conditions however they can be recollections or feelings too.

At that point consider the impacts of the circumstance on your feelings and practices. What were your contemplations, and what social did you take? Offer your sentiments. Pick and circle the one impression or feeling which appeared to be the greatest corresponding to the occurrence. Pause for a minute currently to burrow down and characterize your considerations, perspectives, discernments, or goals in this circumstance. In the event that you experience issues recognizing your feelings, consider what sort of considerations could have added to your sentiments. Pause for a minute to compose these down.

Pick the one that most bother you and circle it. The sorts of considerations that lead to your stress can differ contingent upon how you see overthinking. I clarify basic kinds of musings in the accompanying areas identifying with various sorts of nervousness. Pick your significant parts and work on perceiving emotions that lead to your nervousness.

4.3. Well known examples of Reasoning

Similarly as there are run of the mill examples of on edge considerations, unsurprising examples of the sorts of musings you have contingent upon your specific stress is additionally famous. The accompanying areas depict some basic examples of thought for every one of the nervousness issue we've talked about. In light of your specific side effects of stress, you might need to focus just on those areas which identify with you.

EXTRAORDINARY FEAR

People with extraordinary fear participate in unhelpful examples of reasoning which add to their stress. In the event that you fear flying, you may overestimate a plane's likelihood of slamming and be careful about indications of mechanical disappointment. In the event that you have an insect fear you can overestimate the hazard and outcomes of gnawing. Claustrophobia can make you question your capacity to adapt in a kept space. Contemplations in a particular fear commonly focus on conceivable outcomes of "imagine a scenario were.

A few instances of normal fear musings include:

- Imagine a scenario in which the lift links break and the lift crashes.
- Imagine a scenario in which I lose control of this divider, and perplex myself.
- Imagine a scenario in which the snake comes out of its storeroom and assaults me.

Think about an ongoing circumstance where you've felt stress or thought. Distinguish sentiments you may have had that could have prompted your nervousness.

SUMMED UP STRESS ISSUE

In the event that you have Stray you may feel day by day restless, overestimating the likelihood of the most exceedingly terrible occurring. Potentially this concern reaches out to all parts of your life, including family, funds, business, wellbeing, and ties. You despite everything have sentiments of "imagine a scenario in which" and are condemning of yourself, or feel incapable to adapt.

You may have considerations like this:

- Imagine a scenario in which I get into a mishap.
- Imagine a scenario in which I can't carry out this responsibility once more.
- Consider the possibility that I'm burdened with a horrendous sickness.
- What occurs in the event that I fail?
- I will lose my employment on the off chance that I don't find an ideal line of work assessment.
- Simply need to guarantee things go easily.
- All choices should be thought of so I can guarantee a decent outcome.

Indeed, even idea about your feelings of thought. You may believe you will get frantic with a lot of stress. Then again, you may feel hesitant to surrender your concern, as though it is some way or another ensuring you. You may experience issues enduring disarray, and overthinking may appear to be productive to you—as though you attempt to fix what's going on.

On the off chance that you have Stray, it might be hard for you to recognize the particular conditions that enact your overthinking, since it appears to be steady. Here's the place your Stress Journal proves to be useful.

Think back and check whether you could recognize explicit conditions where you feel more worried than typical. What had caused your extraordinary nervousness scenes? It is safe to say that you are headed toward work driving on the interstate? Confronted with the chance of advancement to an increasingly responsible position? Holding up in the workplace of the Specialist? Taking care of tabs?

SOCIAL OVERTHINKING DISORDER

Considerations that initiate a social nervousness depend on being decided by others, or feeling like others may see your stress. In spite of the fact that it might appear as though a circumstance is straightforwardly making your heart pound, your hands to shake, and your brain clear, yet it's the musings you have about the circumstance that is influencing your response.

At the point when it came to open speaking, Tom had musings like, "Everybody's going to perceive how tense I'm," "I'm not going to have the option to keep my hands from shaking and "individuals will get exhausted."

At last, you may have contemplations, for example, these:

- I have not said anything in quite a while. Everyone needs to believe I'm unusual.
- Nobody converses with me. They don't need to like me.

- I can feel everybody taking a gander at me when I go into the room. I generally commit errors before people.
- Everyone believes I'm an awful speaker to the press. I am stressed to such an extent that I realize they can tell.

Return to your stress Journal and depict a circumstance you had felt apprehensive about. Presently, depict the sentiments you had that may have prompted the manner in which you felt at that point. Record the episode, your passionate outcome and your emotions.

Frenzy Issue

On the off chance that you have alarm issue, you're conceivably captivating in calamitous speculation—in which the issues of "imagine a scenario in which" begin turning crazy. You might be concerned that the indications of your overthinking demonstrate something is genuinely amiss with you, and you may likewise be stressed that others may think you are having an open fit of anxiety.

Here are a few instances of frenzy issue anxious musings:

- I sense that I will go insane.
- I generally should be in control. I can't let anybody alarm come to see me.
- My heart pulsates so hard, it is by all accounts a respiratory failure.
- I feel so dizzy and sluggish. I figure I would swoon.

Return to your Overthinking Journal and investigate the frenzy activating conditions. Would you be able to recollect any sentiments you had at that point? Note the circumstance, and depict your key idea and response.

AGORAPHOBIA

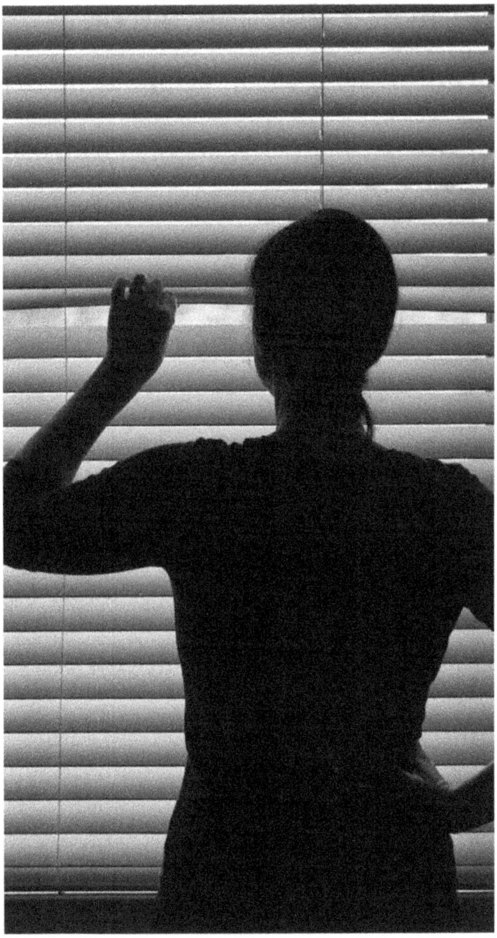

Agoraphobia involves the thought of having a fit of anxiety that others will perceive, or it will be hard to escape from. Musings sustaining this type of overthinking thusly incorporate those of pondering what might unfurl on the off chance that you had a fit of anxiety openly.

The following are two instances of such reflections.

- Imagine scenarios where I lose adjust and have an open frenzy issue where everybody can see.
- In the event that I begin having a fit of anxiety, I won't ever have the option to leave.

Return to your Journal on overthinking. Would you be able to perceive a condition that has caused agoraphobic frenzy suppositions? Record the circumstance, the key contemplations and the result.

4.4. Uncovering the Center Convictions

The recognizable proof procedure of your center convictions isn't vastly different from what you've just done. It is tied in with growing the musings you depicted to their basic topic. One method for getting to those center convictions is to ask you, "What does that mean?" In response to your negative reasoning
Your center conviction is the incredible thought which drives different feelings of trepidation. Likewise, your different feelings of thought tap it, and invigorate it more. In case you're similar to Tom, and you believe you're sufficiently bad, individuals' musings disliking you fit in that center conviction.

CHAPTER FIVE: BREAKING AWAY FROM THE HABITS OF NEGATIVE THINKING

In the last part, we distinguished negative musings that lead to your nervousness and made an arrangement to utilize your Overthinking Journal and the Perceiving Considerations structure to work on perceiving those contemplations. We additionally started investigating center convictions toward the finish of the last part the fundamental subjects at the focal point of your negative musings, which are likewise reinforced by them.

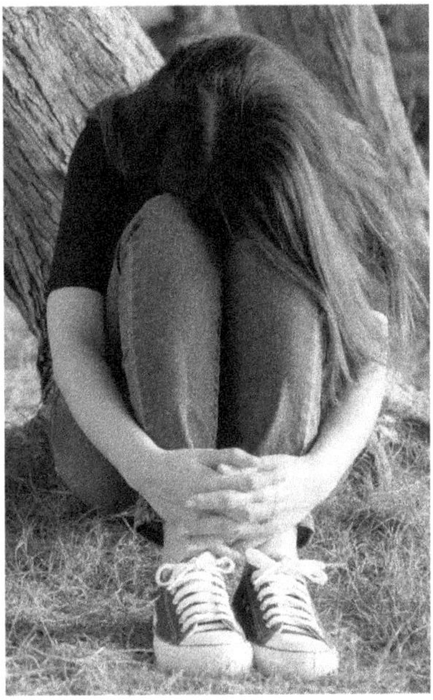

We will characterize your own basic beliefs in this part, and figure out how to break your negative examples of reasoning. We will investigate your contemplations in the part, and challenge their precision.

Now I might want you to return to your last week's Stress Journal and Thought Recognizable proof structures. Pick one case, and record your recorded contemplations. We will look at these thoughts as we progress through this section and perceive how well they are holding up to examination.

5.1. For what reason would we say we are holding tight to convictions?

At the point when you look at your considerations and convictions, you'll likely discover detours to relinquish the individuals who end up being bogus or unhelpful. For the most part talking, there are three reasons why you may adhere to unhelpful or deceptions:

Initially, you may imagine that there is legitimacy to what you accept and that relinquishing that conviction would be a shallow method to handle your concern.

You want to be convinced that your conviction isn't right, thus far, on the side of that speculation, you have not seen evidence.

Also, you may realize that your conviction is bogus on a consistent level, yet it despite everything influences you in a passionate manner. For instance, in some way or another you may realize that attempting to accomplish flawlessness in each social circumstance isn't intelligent, however the outlook endures and causes you trouble.

At long last, ideologies are here and there just kept clumsy. You realize your conviction isn't right, and it no longer heavily affects your feelings—yet you can't release it any longer. Those feelings are mind-numbingly repetitive in your brain playing ambient melodies. For instance, on the off chance that you have alarm issue, you may coherently understand that your side effects don't infer you're having a cardiovascular failure; however it's consistently the idea that is introducing itself. Think about the circumstance you are in. Would it be advisable for you to clutch contemplations since you unequivocally accept they are valid? Are there any considerations that you don't accept totally any more, yet at the same time aim trouble? Do you have on edge considerations that are unadulterated negative behavior patterns? Glance back at the considerations you've revealed in the past segment and miracle why you're staying with them. Record your considerations.

5.2. Six snappy approaches to oversee negative reasoning

Throughout the years, a method called "thought halting," which incorporates pulling an elastic band or making some other move at whatever point you have a negative idea, has pulled in some consideration. The thinking behind this system is that you're ready to prepare yourself to dodge negative reasoning.

Tragically, it can do the converse and lead to expanded negative reasoning, on the off chance that you remain continually cautious of mistaken idea. The objective ought not to be to expel every single negative idea yet rather to figure out how to all the more likely oversee them. Like irritating spring up promotions on numerous sites, negative musings will consistently come up—yet you don't have to focus on them.

The following are six basic methods for really dealing with your negative reasoning.

1. Only one inclination. Imprint your considerations as a minor idea and not a reality.
   Let yourself know, for instance, "I'm believing I'm reluctant to give my associates this introduction," which assists with separating yourself and be progressively objective.

2. Diminish the intensity of an Inclination. Envision voicing your idea in a clever voice or singing it to the tune of a melody for youngsters. In this sense, your reasoning will appear to be silly and its capacity will decrease.
3. Spot yourself positive. Neutralize your negative speculation in a proactive way.

Make a rundown of your victories at work on the off chance that you are worried about coming up short at your particular employment.

4. Assess the reasoning. Ask yourself, "Is this idea genuine, significant or supportive?" Distinguishing unhelpful contemplations will empower you to separate yourself from them.
5. Separate yourself from thought. Envision composing the idea on a bit of paper, and sending it away in a container as a message. Watch while your concerns coast away.
6. Put aside some an opportunity to consider. Put aside an opportunity to manage alarming emotions later on, so you can release them in the present.

5.3. Negative Idea Challenge

Presently I need you to consider the circumstance you found in this section before. Pick the one idea that in that circumstance appeared to give you the most thinking – we consider this the "hard" thought, or the one that causes your passionate response. At that point utilize the Difficult Your Musings strategy beneath to discover realities for and against your thinking, assess your idea's exactness, and concoct an increasingly practical other option.

Here are a couple of inquiries you have to pose to yourself when rounding out the structure:

- Would you say you are certain your musings are valid?
- Taking a gander at occasions throughout your life, what evidence is there to support your reasoning?
- What evidence does the opposite demonstrate valid?
- Do you exaggerate the risk?
- Is there one more clarification?
- Does the entire picture consider your musings?

AT THE POINT WHEN MUSINGS ARE EXACT

Since there isn't sufficient proof to help your case, an increasingly balanced clarification can rather be subbed. This is substantial if, for instance, you fear flying, in light of the fact that the real danger of a plane slamming is extremely little.

Are there times where perspectives and feelings might be exact? Perhaps you think your hands shake with companions when having supper in an eatery. You could discover in looking at the proof that your hands shook frequently in this sort of circumstance previously. In this situation, your instinct is by all accounts exact—the possibility your hands would shake is likely high. Let yourself know, if my reasoning is correct, what is the direst outcome imaginable? In the event that you concur that when you go out to a café your hands will shake a bit, yet realize that in the event that it happens it's anything but a calamity, at that point that idea will lose a portion of its quality.

You'll presumably discover in cases like this that the outcomes you anticipate are not as awful as you thought. On the off chance that your enthusiastic reaction to transpiring is messed up with regards to the occasion, it may be the case that the reasoning affirms a wrong center conviction.

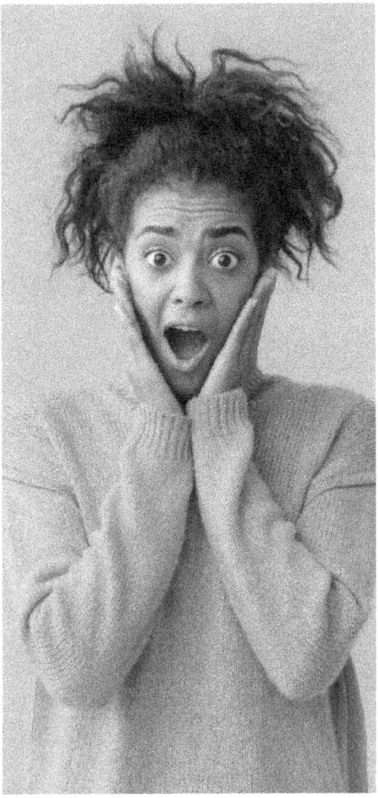

The center confidence for this situation might be that you should never show thought in others' organization. Think about the circumstance you are in. Is it true that you were terrified of episodes with an incredibly low possibility of occurring? In the event that you are frightful of things that are probably going to happen, is the outcome a disaster or would you be able to figure out how to adapt?

The manner in which we decipher occasions, conditions and what others state and do relates legitimately to our own encounters. Such recognitions construct suppositions about us, about others and about the world. Also, our center conviction framework is the thing that permits us to comprehend what we are encountering. On the off chance that your center convictions are negative, altering them can be the impetus for dependable, positive change.

5.4. Changing Center Convictions

Unhelpful reasoning regularly requires a bogus impression of a circumstance which can prompt expanded nervousness.

CREATING OPTIONS

Presently I need you to finish a Graph of Center Conviction for your own condition. Identify a center conviction and the fundamental negative considerations which have advanced out of that center conviction. You may even have a few center convictions that various arrangements of musings hold. Incorporate however many of the charts of center conviction as could be allowed to characterize the fundamental subjects of your negative reasoning. On the off chance that you experience difficulty getting to the inside, ask yourself inquiries about your negative contemplations, similar to "I'm not catching this' meaning?" And "What'd not be right with that? As a result of something named "affirmation predisposition," the center convictions are held. We will in general search for proof that affirms our feelings and excuse proof that is against them. I need you to record the center faith in the space underneath that you might want to scrutinize the most. Discover then any experiences you have had that are conflicting to your center conviction.

For example, if your center conviction is that you're futile, you could compose things like "I'm a given parent," or "I'm chipping in my time." In light of the realities that conflict with your conviction, produce another, increasingly sane and sensible conviction. What might you say to another in a similar spot as you? Your new elective conviction, for instance, could be "I am a commendable individual."

USING POSITIVE ATTESTATIONS

The unhelpful or broken center convictions can be addressed with positive insistences. Attestations are little proclamations which you rehash recorded as a hard copy or verbally to yourself. The following are a few proposals for composing and utilizing positive attestations.

It makes them simpler to review, and shows progress in the present as opposed to later on eventually. It is smarter to state "I am quiet" than "I can resist the urge to panic even in troublesome circumstances," or "I should resist the urge to panic." Utilize positive words. "I remain quiet when conversing with outsiders" is better than "I'm not terrified when addressing outsiders." Thoughtful words have an approach to stay with you in any event, when stated adversely, so it is sensible to utilize positive words.

Be genuine. The most grounded explanations are about enhancements that you need to find in your life and that you're willing to progress in the direction of such issues just like "a positive open speaker," or "I'm figuring out how to be a sure open speaker." Each morning, write down your insistences in a journal or spot them on stickers in places you see each day, for example, your washroom mirror or PC screen.

Do a chronicle. Leave 6 to 11 seconds between each sentence so you'll have the opportunity to gradually process what you're stating. When daily, tune in to the account. Do this for one month. Hear it out while you clean the house, drive your vehicle, or nod off.

While it might feel awkward or clumsy from the outset to make statements about yourself that you don't completely accept, it ought to get increasingly ordinary with time. It resembles the well-known axiom "counterfeit it till you do it." The equivalent can be said about how you're conversing with you.

5.5. Normal center convictions

The center convictions speak to what you, others and your general surroundings think about yourself. They are the entirety of your negative considerations and are influenced by your encounters, the earth of the young, society, convictions, confidence and current conditions. Center convictions regularly have ideas of vulnerability, unviability, or uselessness. Regularly, they embrace the "I am" or "I need to" model. The following are some basic fundamental beliefs for each kind of stress. You can skirt parts that are not applicable to the kind of overthinking you're feeling.

EXPLICIT FEAR

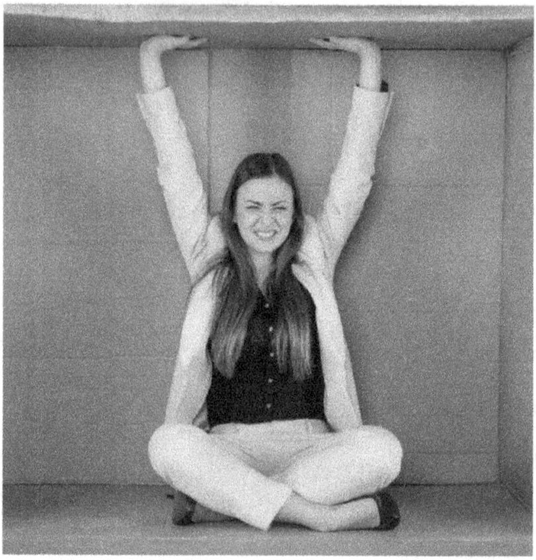

Claustrophobia may leave you in the feeling that on the off chance that you ride in a lift you're going to freeze and go insane.

Fundamental beliefs like these can be tried for their exactness in like manner fear. What is the probability that a snake is venomous or assaulting you? How likely is it that riding a lift would make you go insane?

In the event that you have a specific fear, consider what basic beliefs your negative musings might be to keep up. Archive your musings.

SOCIAL OVERTHINKING ISSUE

One normal idea in the state of social stress is that you are sufficiently bad. Some of the time, this conviction may develop because of a strong, ejective, or overprotective parent, or negative friend encounters.

Some normal center convictions about social stress include:

- I'm futile (dumb, exhausting, unlikeable, ugly, undesirable, and so on.).

- I'm not taking tally.
- I'm not sufficiently acceptable.
- I must have others affirm.
- Another person rates me.

In case you're reluctant to converse with outsiders, it's most likely in light of the deception that you think they'll see you dull or unlikable. At the point when you're apprehensive about open talking, you may feel like you're not a sufficient speaker. As a rule, any occurrence where you wind up in the organization of others may have the inclination you have to gauge up here and there. On the off chance that your center conviction is that you should consistently have another person's endorsement, would you be able to turn that around and inquire as to whether that is pragmatic or accommodating?

Locate the central qualities that lead to the negative idea designs, regardless of whether you have social nervousness. Record your musings.

FRENZY ISSUE AND AGORAPHOBIA

I have assembled alarm issue and agoraphobia as they seem to speak to comparable center convictions. Here are a few instances of center convictions you may have related to freeze issue and agoraphobia:

- I will go insane.
- I am insufficient.
- I am down and out.
- I can't adapt to that.
- I feel powerless.
- I don't have to show shortcoming.
- Consistently must be in charge.

Regularly the center conviction of frenzy issue and agoraphobia is that you generally must be in control and not show shortcoming. Going to open spots is hazardous because of the danger of having a fit of anxiety and not having the option to get away from the circumstance. In the event that this lines up with you, at that point it might be useful to inquire as to why you trust you ought to never be helpless.

In the event that you have crucial convictions about frenzy issue or agoraphobia, record them.

SUMMED UP STRESS ISSUE

Center convictions in like manner overthinking issue mirror a worldwide topic that is a dubious, risky spot and a requirement for power. Unsteady conditions in the adolescence and guardians with excessively elevated standards may likewise lay the preparation for these sorts of center convictions. The following are a few instances of Stray center convictions:

- Awful things are going to occur.
- The world is a jeopardized zone.
- I must be sure of acceptable outcomes.

For summed up overthinking issue, when you thought the obscure, center convictions are regularly connected to a requirement for affirmation. For this situation it might be useful to ask yourself comparative inquiries as in like manner fears—what is the probability that your feelings of thought will really worked out as expected?

OK concur with any of the center convictions related with a summed-up nervousness issue? Provided that this is true, get your emotions.

5.6. Assembling Everything

It's an ideal opportunity to begin constructing your new idealistic center convictions since you've set up your negative center convictions and think of increasingly objective other options. I need you to keep an information log throughout the following section which records proof that underpins your new center convictions. For instance, if your new conviction is "I am sure," during a conversation you may report the second you communicated an alternate conclusion. Track these exercises at the rear of this book on the lined pages. Just observe the new conviction and afterward record any cases that underlie it.

FEAR OF GOING CRAZY OR LOSING CONTROL

A typical factor is the thought of going crazy or losing control of numerous nervousness issue. You may fear being mortified or being removed in an emergency vehicle, for instance. While stress that cause manifestations that make you believe you will lose control, the inclination will in general go back and forth with your nervousness level. Then again, on the off chance that you were truly losing contact with the real world, you would be bound to have little information on what was going at.

At the point when you have a feeling that you're losing contacts with the current second, attempt to concentrate on your environment. Notice the blue sky, peeping flying creatures, or the smell of someone's scent—whatever brings your concentration once more into the present.

SELF-DAMAGE

Be keeping watch for self-damage in the coming week while you move in the direction of scrutinizing your fundamental beliefs and ruinous considerations. It might feel alarming to relinquish old perspectives and you might be ending up slipping go into old propensities, particularly during times of pressure. Make certain to take continuous measures towards progress to keep this from occurring, make little strides when you feel overpowered in conditions and be aware of your own evasion. For instance, if your past propensity was to over and over call a friend or family member for consolation when you were worried by your interests, discover choices that can likewise help assuage your pressure. Consider about what a sensible individual may be doing in a similar circumstance. Have a go at taking a walk or practicing in the rec center as an elective technique to depend a lot on others around you for consolation in the event that you have an intense day at work. It isn't at all improper to contact friends and family however to stop continually doing as such.

It's additionally imperative to be vigilant about shirking as you step towards increasingly hopeful center convictions. In the event that you have alarm issue, for instance, you may be working on a supposition that you can adapt to on edge emotions. On the off chance that that feels overwhelming, you may begin staying away from conditions that you thought could cause a fit of anxiety. Rather, attempt to go about as though the center conviction had just been substantial. What might you do on the off chance that you realized you could adapt similarly just as others?

Is it true that you were stressed over falling go into negative reasoning and center negative convictions? Record any issues you anticipate and how you will manage if those issues emerge.

CPSIA information can be obtained
at www.ICGtesting.com
Printed in the USA
BVHW071622300421
606209BV00005B/541

9 781802 534252